The Magic of Aloe Vera

Dueep J Singh
Natural Remedy Series
Mendon Cottage Books

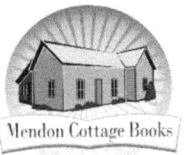

JD-Biz Publishing

Download Free Books!

http://MendonCottageBooks.com

Our books are available at

1. Amazon.com
2. Barnes and Noble
3. Itunes
4. Kobo
5. Smashwords
6. Google Play Books

Download Free Books!

http://MendonCottageBooks.com

Table of Contents

Knowing more about Aloe Vera 5

Grow Aloe Vera In Your Garden 8

How to use the Aloe Vera leaf? 12

Aloe Vera In Ancient Medicine 13

Diabetes 14

How to make Desi Ghee (clarified butter), to use in making up Aloe Vera ointments 15

Arthritis 16

Liver Tonic 16

Sprain remedy 17

Aloe Vera in Cooking 18

Traditional Aloe Vera Curry 20

Aloe Vera as a beauty product 22

Your own alphahydroxy acids 24

How to make Rose water (Gulab Jal) 25

Exfoliating Aloe Vera Facial Scrub 26

Herbal Shampoo with Aloe Vera 26

Face wash powder 28

PH balanced skin toner 28

Conclusion 29

Author Bio.. 30

Publisher.. 41

Knowing more about Aloe Vera

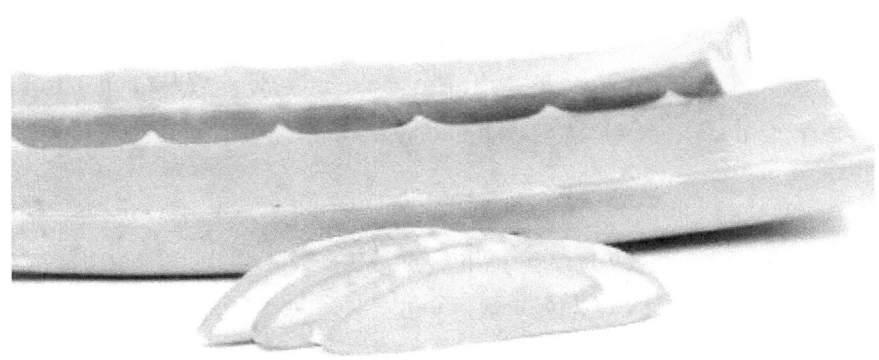

As a child, growing up in wild woody jungles and in mountain regions, where one had to continuously fight against the encroachment of the wild woods trying to take over one's gardens, I noticed that some plants grew only in our gardens, while others grew only in the woods.

One such garden plant was the Aloe Vera, which was a must on every gardener's gardening list. It was always grown in a sunny area, outside the kitchen, and watered once every four or five days, or when one remembered to water it. This green plant was not very attractive to someone who liked flowers around them in their strictly regimented and well disciplined borders and beds. But it was extremely attractive to all those who wanted to know all about the medicinal qualities of this bitter tasting mucilageous succulent.

Also, it did not need lots of fussing to grow. Once it was planted, it flourished as an everlasting perennial

Aloe Vera has been used for millenniums in ancient medicine recipes and remedies, down the ages and in different ancient civilizations. There was a time when it was supposed to grow over large areas in the wild in North Africa, Morocco and other regions around the Sahara desert region, which was once covered with green forests. But as the now desert area began to dry, this plant started dying out in the wild.

Every ancient civilization's medical teachers would tell their students, "Do not underestimate the power of the humble Aloe Vera, my son, because this plant under your kitchen window is going to keep you and your family healthy. Your children shall never suffer from any grave disease internally or externally, your wife shall remain everlastingly beautiful and you shall live a happy and prosperous life, as long as you know all about the benefits of this magical plant." No wonder, it was considered to be a wonder plant by ancient herbalists and medicine men.

Women knew all about its skin rejuvenating quantities millenniums ago, and I am sure that any ancient Egyptian queen would have told her tire woman – are you making up a skin beautifying remedy for me, with asses milk and spices and attar of roses? Add some Aloe Vera to it so that I may look like a goddess for mankind to worship." Cleopatra did that and so did Nefertiti.

This book is going to tell you all about the magic of aloe Vera, its beneficial health and beauty properties, the use of Aloe Vera in ancient medicine, and also how you can use it in cooking. The scooped up inner portion of an Aloe Vera leaf is bitter in taste. That is why it was considered to be on par with

Neem in its beneficial qualities in ancient Indian, Egyptian, Chinese, Greek, and Persian medicine. Its main purpose was to heal, soothe and rejuvenate. They tell us tales of a very beautiful Mogul princess who found herself badly burned because an oil lamp got upset over her delicate skin. Now, being an aristocrat, she did not run screaming out of her chambers, though her slave girls went into hysterical and apoplexy mode, which was their way of not dealing with reality. She just walked out into her garden, and plucked some Aloe Vera leaves, scooped up the mucilage and applied it all over her burns. Aloe Vera healed her body and turmeric got rid of the burn scars. This is the real story of how medical knowledge learned from her ancestors helped Princess Jahan Ara, the daughter of Emperor Shah Jahan – the Emperor who built the Taj Mahal – keep herself beautiful and young looking throughout her life.

Believe it or not, this plant was called the plant of immortality by Egyptians and was praised in their papyri in *sixteen century BC.* That was because the Egyptians used the Aloe Vera pulp, not only to beautify their skins, and keep themselves younger looking, but they carried a mixture of bread mold [we know it as penicillin] and Aloe Vera gel into their battlefields to treat the wounds incurred in war.

So, if you have Aloe Vera growing right under your kitchen wall, well, you do not have to spend lots of money in making cosmetics made up of Aloe Vera gel. You are going to get plenty of information on how you can make beauty products and lotions, right here.

So now you know all about this versatile natural healer, it is time to grow it in your garden.

Grow Aloe Vera In Your Garden

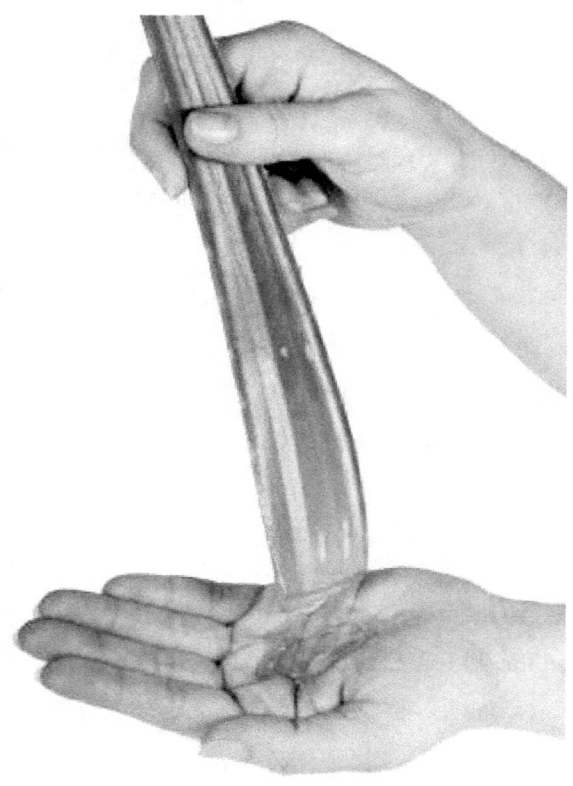

Now seriously, here am I talking about growing Aloe Vera in my garden, when I know that a majority of us live in flats cooped up in cities far away from them thar wide open spaces where the deer and the antelope play. But that does not mean that you cannot grow an Aloe Vera potted plant right in a room where there is plenty of sun. However, if you happen to belong to one of those unfortunate minorities cooped up in a cage, where there is no sun and how do you grow a sun loving potted plant there, never despair. As long as your Aloe gets 8 to 10 hours of light every day, even from a bulb, it will think itself basking in the sun.

There was an Aloe Vera plant flourishing in our chicken coop of a sunless office, some years ago. We normally forgot to water it, but because it was a succulent it did not mind not being over watered. Besides, it knew that when we remembered to water it, we never drowned it in our conscientious and a bit disconcerting Water Our Poor Plant rush towards it. That was because our coffee mugs full of water were quite small water container holders. I think it enjoyed the noise and bustle and attention. Also because the tube lights were always on, it did not mind not being in the sun.

Nevertheless, even though this plant is a houseplant, it would like you to plant it in a place where it can get easy access to indirect sun.

Prepare a pot mixture with plenty of organic fertilizer. Now let me admit something. Whenever I decide to pot a plant, I add plenty of organic fertilizer got from the nearby farms. That is ordinary dried cow dung. These cow dung cakes have been used through millenniums in the East, as fuel and as organic fertilizer. I saw one of our gardeners mixing some ordinary tobacco in the soil he prepared for bulbs and flower plants. He said that that kept away pests in the soil. He also used to spray plants with a tobacco – water spray to kill off all the pests.

Plant it in a wide container. Make sure that there is adequate drainage, because the little bit of water left unabsorbed in the soil is going to cause root rot.

Sorry, Aloe Vera is definitely not going to survive in a place where there is a cold frost. The mucilage content in the leaves "freeze. "That is because they are 95% water. So, the moment the temperature makes you feel shivery, bring your plant inside.

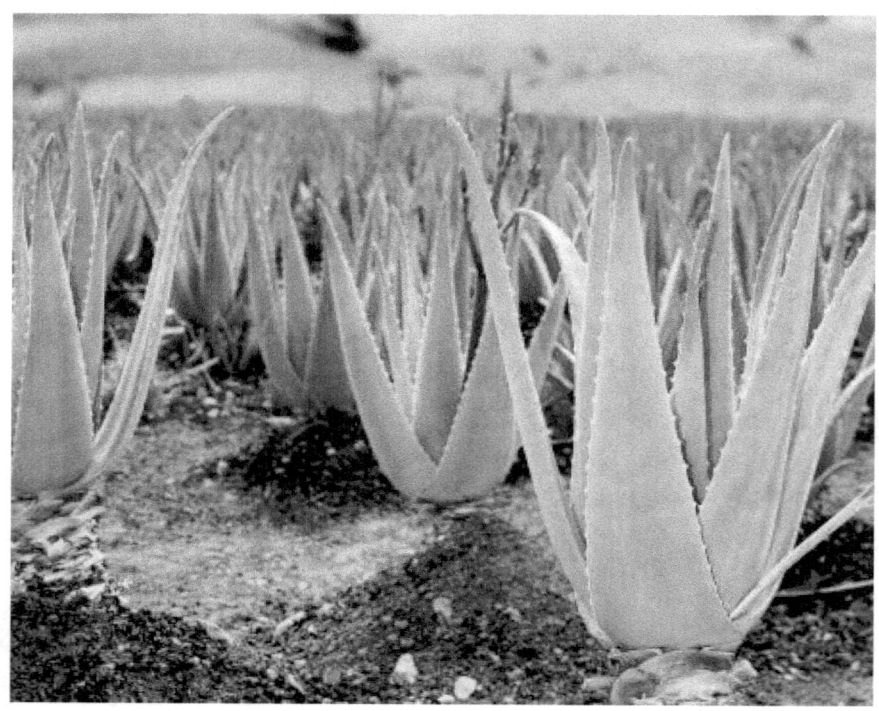

Leaf rot and root rot are common Aloe Vera problems, which are normally caused when water is allowed to remain stagnant in the pot without adequate drainage.

In the East, terra-cotta – baked pots are normally used to plant this succulent, because the baked clay absorbs all that extra water. So if you can plant it in a clay – baked pot, so much the better. I saw containers made out of cement, a couple of weeks ago, and though they were a very attractive addition to your gardens or to your rooms I knew that cement containers are definitely not good water absorbers. Also, I am rather sanguine   about whether these containers are eco-friendly or not, because cement is normally made up of limestone, clay, sand and shale. I may be mistaken but I have never seen a really good plant growth in areas which are rich in limestone. Unless of course they are limestone tolerant like Acacia and eucalyptus.

How to use the Aloe Vera leaf?

I would not suggest breaking the Aloe Vera leaf from its tip. That means the leaf is not going to grow again. Instead, you are going to see some yellowish sort of sap coming out from the injured portion, which is the aloe Vera's way to heal the damage. However, you cut any place along the leaf, it is going to regrow. You can try this experiment. Remove a piece of Aloe Vera from the leaf with the help of a sharp knife. Hold it by the tough outer skin side and rub the mucilage gel material right on your skin. Do not rub any leaf portion which has a yellow sap oozing on it. This sap is not going to benefit your skin any. Or you can cut more mature leaves and stand them upright on a saucer. This is going to drain away the yellow sap. Then cut the serrated edges, as well as the spiky tip. Lay the leaf on a flat surface and make a cut in the middle of the leaf as if you are filleting a fish. Scoop out the gel, from inside the leaf and collected in a bowl. This gel is green in color, and this is what you are going to be using on your skin, or in medical preparations.

When I was a child, I spent a major part of my time breaking off the leaves and squeezing them.

That was because I fell a prey very often to cuts, wounds, sprains and bruises. The gel used to come pouring out just like a jelly. This jelly was then rubbed on directly on the wound. This was definitely not the major curative part of the plant. The innermost mucilage is the most potent and healing part of the plant. Make sure that you do not have any sort of yellow sap polluting the pure green mucilage/gel content.

Aloe Vera In Ancient Medicine

Even though researchers are subjecting this versatile plant to scientific study, because they would rather not see the evidence of their own eyes or of time-tested remedies being used down the ages since ancient times, but would prefer to waste precious time and money on getting some statistics which were already known, well, that is their prerogative. I am surprised to see some knowledgeable researcher coming up with a statement like "There is not enough scientific evidence to support Aloe Vera for any of its other uses …" (*National Center for Complementary and Alternative Medicine (NCCAM)*). Well, like I said, time and money…

Naturally, they will not take into view the knowledge that Aloe Vera has been used in alternative medicine, in Japan, China, Mexico, Egypt, India, Persia, and other ancient civilizations for millenniums. They would rather waste weeks testing out human guinea pigs against their own chemical-based drugs, and hiding the fact that natural remedies are much better alternatives than chemical drugs any day anywhere, anytime. And also, there are some pharmaceuticals and artificially manufactured flavoring companies out there against alternative medicine remedies which do not want to publicize the fact that Aloe Vera is being used as a natural food flavoring which has been approved by the FDA. Well, I go by the knowledge written by Pliny the elder -who died in the eruption of Vesuvius, 79 BC, while trying to leave Herculaneum and Pompeii by sea- in his Natural History about this magical healing plant. Also, in ancient Ayurveda, this plant is used to treat a number of skin diseases, because of the presence of saponin which is an anti-microbial agent.

Diabetes

A doctor who suffered from diabetes tried out this experiment of a mixture of Aloe Vera juice along with the bitter gourd juice once a day to control his sugar levels. According to them, this worked wonderfully for him. I do not know whether there is any scientific basis of Aloe Vera helping him, but everybody knows that ancient Indian medicine uses bitter gourd juice to help cure diabetes. A glass full of Aloe Vera and bitter gourd with his lunch was a part of his daily diet. And he says that he feels more energetic and healthier.

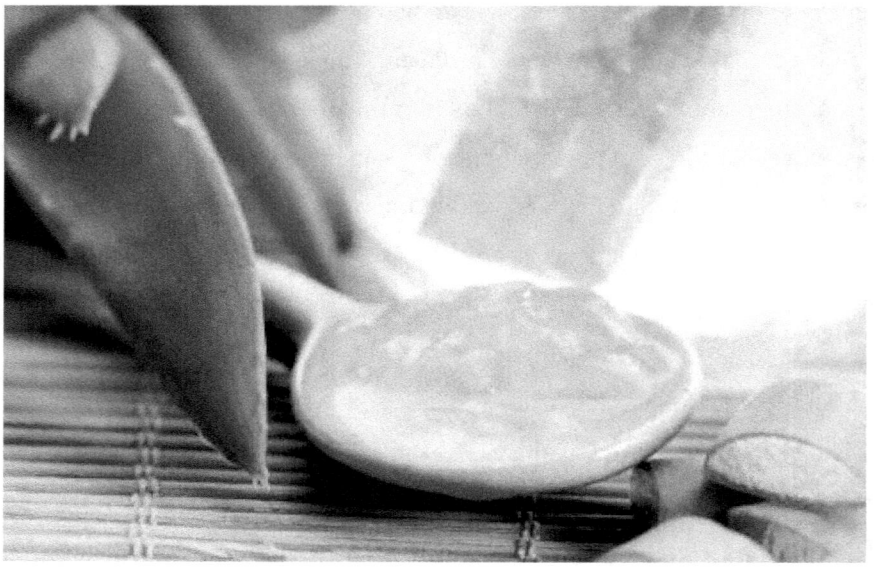

Too much oral ingestion of Aloe Vera may cause you to suffer from diarrhea, because Aloe Vera has been used as a laxative, along with castor seeds in the East for ages. Also, if you eat too much of this plant, you may suffer from nausea, a dry mouth and a headache. Well, nausea, and dry mouth is the logical side effect to something so strong. I find the same side effect if I drink neem juice which is equally beneficial, but which is equally strong and causes an equally bad tasting dry mouth. You may want to try some fresh orange juice over this to balance the electrolytes. In India, it is normally chased up with a tablespoon of concentrated clarified butter – desi ghee. That prevents any potential harmful side effects through drinking large quantities of this normally health giving juice.

Many kitchens in the East have a mixture of clarified butter – Aloe Vera gel – turmeric in glass bottles. That is because cooks consider it to be an excellent healing mixture to cope with kitchen disasters like Burns and scalds

How to make Desi Ghee (clarified butter), to use in making up Aloe Vera ointments.

Start collecting cream from your daily milk supply. 6 to 8 days, will give you enough of cream to make Desi ghee. Heat the milk cream, and you are going to find it melting into Desi ghee. The leftover sediment is delicious, when spread on Indian breads, Pita breads, or over any spicy dish.

Villagers traditionally make Desi ghee in Asia by adding yogurt to the cream for a week or so. They intend to turn it into buttermilk, fresh butter and Desi ghee by churning. This turning process has three stages. Add water to the yoghurt cream mixture and you get buttermilk and butter. Heat the butter and you are going to get Desi ghee.

Remember to remove the sediment from the top, when you store this Desi ghee in airtight glass bottles. The sediment is delicious on breads with honey. One tablespoonful of this highly concentrated powerful oil spread on every meal surface, including vegetables, pulses and beans - every available visible surface - and eaten every day is considered to be the reason why so many people stay healthy in the villages of Asia. This is, of course, supported with plenty of hard physical work throughout the day.

Arthritis

Treat arthritis by massaging a mixture of Aloe Vera pulp in warm mustard oil, all over the affected area. You can also extract the pulp, heat it with any oil – coconut oil, wheat germ oil and olive oil – place it on a piece of cotton and allow it to "foment" the painful area. This is going to alleviate the pain.

Liver Tonic

This **liver tonic** was told to me by an ancient Shaman. He says that he is ninety-seven years old, but he lies. I am sure that he is not less than 120 or even more, going by his wrinkles and his old wise eyes. But he has really dark hair, because he eats 50 g/ml Aloe Vera pulp with milk every day without fail. [A little less than 2 tablespoons.] He says, that that stopped the graying process. Well, I will start doing that when I reach my 60s.

 Also, he made this **liver tonic** for me, and here is the recipe –

Take 1 kg of Aloe Vera pulp. Add 50 g of lemon juice, 5 g of Indian gooseberry powder, 5 g of powdered ginger, and 50 g of pure rock salt. Mix them all together, place them in a glass jar and allow this tonic to ripen in the sun for 10 to 15 days. Now every morning take 3 teaspoons of this liquid without fail to tone up your liver. This is 15 mL. **1 tablespoon is 30 mL.**

Sprain remedy

This is something which I found out on my own. I am a great fan of aloe Vera. I am also a great fan of turmeric. I am not so great a fan of mustard oil, which is also a great curative, but how it does pong. And that is why some days ago, when I twisted my ankle, [sprain, sprain go away] I tried out this remedy. Take out the pulp of aloe Vera. Add some turmeric powder to it. Heat it on slow heat until the turmeric gets assimilated in the aloe Vera. Allow to cool to lukewarm. Put this paste on a piece of cotton cloth and bind up the sprain. I found the pain lessening on two or three applications, which I did as soon as the mixture had started to cool down. I think this is autosuggestion, or perhaps even the application of hot and cold. You may want to try it. Remember that turmeric stains. So do not apply this mixture when you are sitting on your sofa or on your bed.

Aloe Vera in Cooking

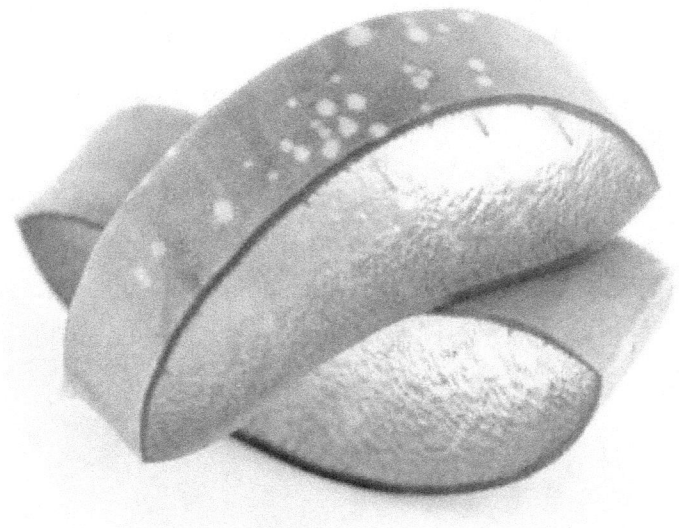

Remember, Aloe Vera in large quantities in cooking may prove to be dangerous to your health, being a laxative. So use it very carefully.

Aloe Vera juice is considered to be a good antioxidant, especially when it is mixed up with other fruit juices like lemon juice, orange juice or any other citrus fruit juice. Ancient doctors believed that a continuous intake of Aloe Vera promoted the circulatory system, purified the blood, helped keep your skin clear, prevented skin diseases like pimples and other skin problems, and maintained the proper healthy balance in your body system.

This is an ancient healthy and rejuvenating remedy, which has been used down the centuries, in the Indian subcontinent, especially when women had to take care of large families. Apart from gooseberry, Aloe Vera was considered to be one of the natural healing plants, which purified your system, both from inside and outside. Just because of its bitter taste, it was considered to be a blood purifier like Neem and bitter gourd.

Now this is a traditional pickle, which you are going to cook in a pickle spice mixture.

You need ten leaves of Aloe Vera, well cleaned, the spikes on the edges removed and the tips cut off.

Now collect the pickle spice mixture – ¼ cup of fenugreek seeds, 1 teaspoon each of powdered chilies, coriander, turmeric, sugar, salt to taste and two hefty pinches of asafoetida, if you want a more Asian taste in your pickles. 2 tablespoons fried Cumin seed and mango powder if you have it around. This last ingredient is going to make this mixture sweet and sour.

My grandmother normally chopped up the peeled leaves' pulps into squares, and then fried all the ingredients together except chilies in a tablespoon of oil. After that she took another frypan and poured in 1 cup of oil. She fried the red chilies and the asafoetida together on slow heat making sure that the chilies were not burned. Burning chilies meant a pungent smoke-filled kitchen, which would bother your family as well as the neighbors. [No wonder, witch doctors in the East always burn chilies in order to scare away evil spirits…]

Now toss the fried Aloe Vera mixture into the chilies and coat all the pieces. Now this is the base of a tasty Aloe Vera pickle. Put this mixture into sterilized glass bottles. I went one step further, I added more oil – I used mustard oil as the base, because that is supposed to make it tastier and supposed to preserve it more – and put this pickle into the sun after I had cooked it. I allowed it to bake in the sun for 5 to 10 days. This allows all the spices to mingle into the Aloe Vera pieces properly.

Do not eat more than one small piece of this pickle, every day. This is good enough to tone up your system.

Traditional Aloe Vera Curry

Now this is something which I learned in Rajasthan, it being a desert area where you could find this succulent which did not bother much about water. And as life is terribly hard for people living in this desert area, they knew how to make the best of any plants, which they found growing in that area, and region.

Chop up the pulp of two Aloe Vera leaves. Boil them with one teaspoonful of salt for three minutes, so that they get pulpy.

Now make a traditional masala of half teaspoon each of fenugreek seeds, aniseeds, coriander powder, red chili powder, any other spice in your larder, cumin seeds, one cardamom, two cloves, pinch of asafoetida and one stick of cinnamon. You may also want to add one spoon of molasses, because in India, we use jaggery to give that sweet taste to the Curry.

This is normally fried in mustard oil. If you are living in the East, you are going to make up the masala, with three tomatoes, 1 cup chopped onions, ginger and garlic. In the West, many people do not like garlic and onions and mustard oil in their masala so they can stay with tomatoes. But I think that half of the fun and the taste of the dish is lost.

Fry the onions, ginger and garlic in your choice of oil – I used mustard. Pungent smelling, but very healthy. Make a brown masala and then slowly add all the powdered spices except chilies. Chilies, then fried in the masala makes the smoke detector in your kitchen howl.

When you get a rich creamy brown gravy, you are going to add the chopped Aloe Vera gel pieces. Fry them on slow heat for a little while, till the spices get assimilated into the vegetable. Now I am going to make a rich gravy with three tablespoonfuls of yogurt. Once you see that the Aloe Vera has been cooked, add the yogurt and fry again, till the liquid becomes a thick and delicious gravy. The Rajasthanis normally eat this with bread, but you can always eat this as an accompaniment to boiled rice. Enjoy.

Why I just said two Aloe Vera leaves? That is because too much of Aloe Vera will have you running to the bathroom, because this is a laxative when taken in large quantities. Besides, when you eat it in a Curry, you are not going to hog all of it in one sitting, are you. This Curry is for the full family. Also, this gel somehow loses its bitterness, when it is cooked in a masala. So enjoy.

Aloe Vera as a beauty product

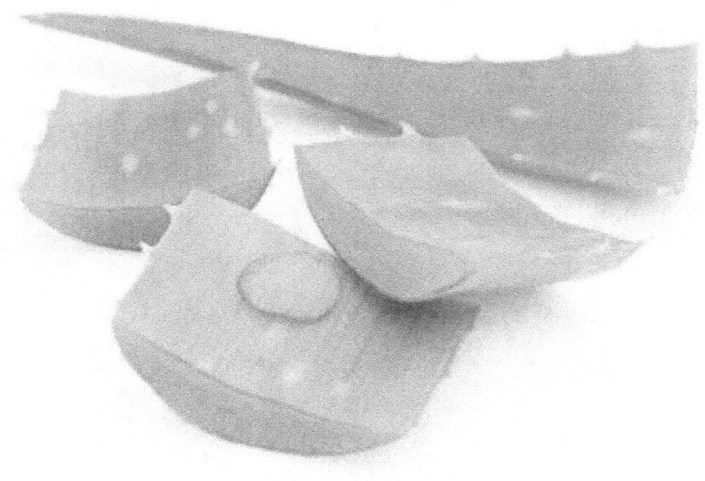

Do not you think it is time for you to stop waiting for miracles promised to you by purveyors of so-called natural expensive beauty products and go in for natural herbal remedies where you can see the results immediately? That is where Aloe Vera comes into its own.

A "Lambarhi"[1] gypsy friend of mine told me that Aloe Vera gel is normally used by South Indian Gypsies as a hair conditioner to prevent and

---

[1] Incidentally, I asked that same friend whether any of her rambling Gypsy ancestors had reached Europe and settled down in an area in Italy called Lombardy, named after their Lambarhi Gypsy clan. I was just being fatuous and was surprised that her answer was – "most probably, yes. Because most of our ancestors went on to Seville in Spain and became famous sword makers for

discourage dandruff in the hair. Just scoop it out, and rub it into your scalp. Well, I know that Aloe Vera is an extremely good moisturizer of your skin, so why should not it not be used to moisturize your scalp? For that, you will need to take out its juice. That can be done very easily, like I explained during the filleting of an Aloe Vera leaf. If you are confronted with any yellowish sublayer under the leaf, you can remove it by putting the leaf in a vinegar water mixture. You will need to scoop out the mucilage from a number of leaves to get enough of material to make some juice. Put all of this gel into a blender and blend into a smooth paste. You can drink this juice. You can also apply this juice as a lemon, Aloe Vera hair conditioner by blending some lemon juice in this mixture.

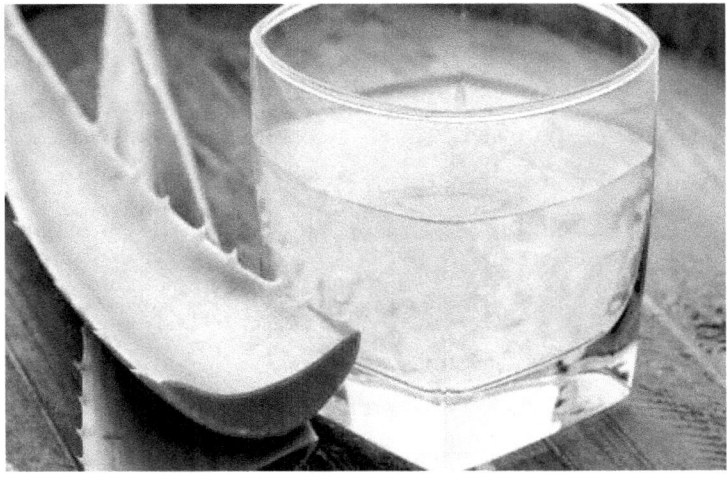

Spanish aristocrats." Those swords were supposed to be rustproof, and made from ancient Gypsy sword making lore which were lost to the Indians in Asia more than 2000 years ago. But I still have an authentic antique heirloom Gypsy iron knife, which has not rusted for the past 400 years or more. These knives are very much in demand and in India, people are always on the lookout for real Gypsies, asking them to make rustproof iron utensils for them.

Here are some natural herbal products, which are going to help you preserve your beauty –

Your own alphahydroxy acids

How many of your expensive cosmetic products have chemical-based alphahydroxy acids shown in the ingredient list? Here are natural hydroxy acids, in the shape of yogurt, lime juice, apple juice and orange juice. Add some Aloe Vera pulp to this mixture. Apply it on your skin. Not only is this going to rejuvenate your skin, but it is also going to moisturize it. You may feel a tingling sensation in the beginning, but this is the affect of natural citric alphahydroxy acids acting on your skin. Do not use this on a broken or damaged skin.

I normally use this as a facial mask. If you get Fullers earth anywhere around you, use this as the most amazing skin tightening and rejuvenating mask. Get cakes of this earth, pounded to a powder. Use it as a facemask mixed with water or rosewater once a week. Avoid the areas around the eyes. Do you know that the beauty professionals and those expenses spas and beauty salons use this product as a main ingredient in your skin toning masks and body scrubs. And you come out feeling so pampered and cherished.

Now that you are using Aloe Vera as a facemask, you may want to add another amazing skin toning liquid to it. In the absence of cream, olive oil, wheat germ oil or fresh milk. This is called Rosewater.

How to make Rose water (Gulab Jal)

Rosewater is normally available in markets at exorbitant prices, but in Asia, anybody with access to the red rose - Rosa Damascena -and a little bit of time enjoys making Rosewater at home. This Rosewater is used in cosmetics, as well as in cookery to impart the flavor of the Rose to your meal as well as to your skin.

Ingredients needed- 1 Cup Rose petals - 12 to 14 flowers.

2 cups water

Lots of ice.

A huge cooking pan - pan number one - with lid in which another pan - pan number two - can be placed comfortably.

Rosewater is just a matter of distillation. Put a wire stand in pan number one, on which you are going to stand the other pan number two. The condensed Rosewater is going to fall into pan number two.

Place the petals at the bottom of the pan number one. Now, cover the petals with water. Place pan number two on the wire stand. Now take the lid and place it upside down on pan number one, thus effectively covering the Rose petals, pan number two and the water. The Rose water is going to condense when you place the blocks and chunks of ice on the inverted lid.

You are going to have a cupful of precious distilled Rosewater, after 25 minutes of slow steaming of the Rose petals.

Precautions - remember to have enough of water to cover the Rose petals. Also, it should not be of such a large quantity, that it displaces the wire stand.

This cooled water is now pure Rosewater. Place it in a sterilized glass bottle. Use it to your heart's content. You may see a little bit of oil swimming over the surface of the water. This is Rose oil, and is even more precious. So if you used lots of petals in a larger pan, you may find even more Rose oil.

This other method is for all those people who use a pressure cooker while cooking food. In fact, it is a common way to cook food in Asian kitchens, instead of using the microwave.

You would need water, petals, a pressure cooker and a long thin pipe which it does not melt, when subjected to heat.

Put the water and the petals in the pressure cooker and cover it. Now cover the thin pipe with wet cloth in order to keep it cool. Attach this pipe on the lid of the pressure cooker where you normally attach the weight. Allow the petals to cook slowly, they seem to build up, go through the cooled pipe and collect in a utensil. I tried this way too, but I find the ice on the lid one easier!

Exfoliating Aloe Vera Facial Scrub

Take two spoons full of oatmeal, half a teaspoonful of Aloe Vera gel, one pinch of salt and one pinch of turmeric. Make a paste using lime juice. Scrub your face gently using this powder. This is considered to be the best exfoliation scrub, removing the dead skin cells, cleansing the pores and rejuvenating dull and tired skin.

Herbal Shampoo with Aloe Vera

Use a mixture of equal parts of powdered gooseberry, and powdered Shikakai. Half this quantity of fenugreek seeds and double the amount of powdered soap nut is going to make a lovely dry mixture. Now add as much of Aloe Vera gel you want added in this mixture, and then make up the shampoo with water. A small quantity of this herbal shampoo is going to keep your hair lovely and lustrous and glowing, and you are also going to find that the graying process diminishes considerably.

Now I am going to tell you all about the herbs I told you in the previous shampoo recipe – the Indian gooseberry is known as Amla- Emblica officianalis. The fruit is made into a powder and use as a beauty product ingredient. It is also considered to be a fruit eaten by the ancients to encourage longevity and prevent aging.

Fenugreek seeds are considered in the East to be promoters of hair growth. Fenugreek is also an important spice in Asian cuisine. The chopped and fried leaves make up a delicious fenugreek and potato dish.

Shikakai – learn more about this herb at http://www.allayurveda.com/shikakai-herb.asp.

This has been used as an Herb from centuries to promote hair growth and to keep the scalp healthy and dandruff free.

Soap nut – even though, we use soap nut for washing our hair, it can also be used to wash all your delicate woolen garments. This has been done down the ages, when delicate garments were not subjected to harsh homemade soaps made of animal fats and lye.

http://betteralive.hubpages.com/hub/How-to-Use-Reetha-or-Soap-Nuts-for-Washing-Hair

All right, confession time – I cheat sometimes by using Ayur shampoos, because I know that they use soap nut, gooseberry, Shikakai extracts and when I am too lazy to make my own shampoos. But I am sure you are going to find the URL given above very helpful. By the way, if you are blonde, light haired or auburn haired, **do not use Shikakai in the herbal shampoo recipe or an iron pot, if you are making your own shampoo, as in the recipe given in the above hub page.** These are to darken your naturally dark hair. Asians steep their shampoos in iron pots because they like dark gleaming hair.

Face wash powder

 I would suggest using Aloe Vera juice every day as a skin tonic and cleanser, as well as a moisturizer. But that should be done, after you have cleaned your face with a little bit of oatmeal and milk. This is a substitute for chemical-based soap. It cleanses without disturbing the natural balance of your skin. Also, it helps to remove black and white heads.

PH balanced skin toner

Add 1 teaspoon of vinegar and a teaspoon of Rosewater to a cup of fresh water. Splash it on your face to feel fresh for hours. Apply a little bit of natural Aloe Vera gel to moisturize your skin.

Last most important beauty tip– nothing works externally if you are not taking care of your internal system. So keep your internal system well irrigated with lots of fresh fruit and vegetable juices, including Aloe Vera juice.

Conclusion

So now that you know all about the magic of Aloe Vera as a medicine, as a green vegetable, which you may want to add to your daily diet, as a provider of a healthy juice, and also as a natural beauty products, why do not you grow it in your house or garden right away. Remember, that this product has been used through centuries by doctors as well as beauties to rejuvenate, heal, cure, and beautify. People are looking into Aloe Vera to cure Psoriasis. I did not find any sort of recipe or remedy in ancient remedy books talking about this plant as a cure for psoriasis, but I know that it is used to cure other skin diseases. So the next time you have suffered an accident in the kitchen or have been exposed to the sun, just snap off a fully grown leaf, scoop out the gel and apply it to the affected area. It is the coolest one!

Author Bio

Dueep Jyot Singh is a Management and IT Professional who managed to gather Postgraduate qualifications in Management and English and Degrees in Science, French and Education while pursuing different enjoyable career options like being an hospital administrator, IT,SEO and HRD Database Manager/ trainer, movie scriptwriter, theatre artiste and public speaker, lecturer in French, Marketing and Advertising, ex-Editor of Hearts On Fire (now known as Solctice) Books Missouri USA, advice columnist and cartoonist, publisher and Aviation School trainer, ex- moderator on Medico.in, banker, student councilor ,travelogue writer … among other things! One fine morning, she decided that she had enough of killing herself by Degrees and went back to her first love -- writing. It's more enjoyable! She already has 48 published academic and 14 fiction- in- different- genre books under her belt.

When she is not designing websites or making Graphic design illustrations for clients who want Walt Disney, Norman Rockwell , JJ Grandville or Hed Kandy type illustrations, she is busy browsing in old bookshops for antique books,-she has a mouthwatering collection of priceless First editions and rare books…including R.L. Stevenson, O.Henry, Dornford Yates, Maurice Walsh, C.N.Williamson, and the crown of her collection- Dickens "The Old Curiosity Shop," and so on… Just call her "Renaissance Woman" - collecting herbal remedies, making one of a kind creations in Irish Crochet and Aran knitting, acting like Universal Helping Hand/Agony Aunt, or escaping to her dear mountains for a bit of exploring, collecting herbs and plants , trekking, and rappelling.

Check out some of the other JD-Biz Publishing books

Gardening Series on Amazon

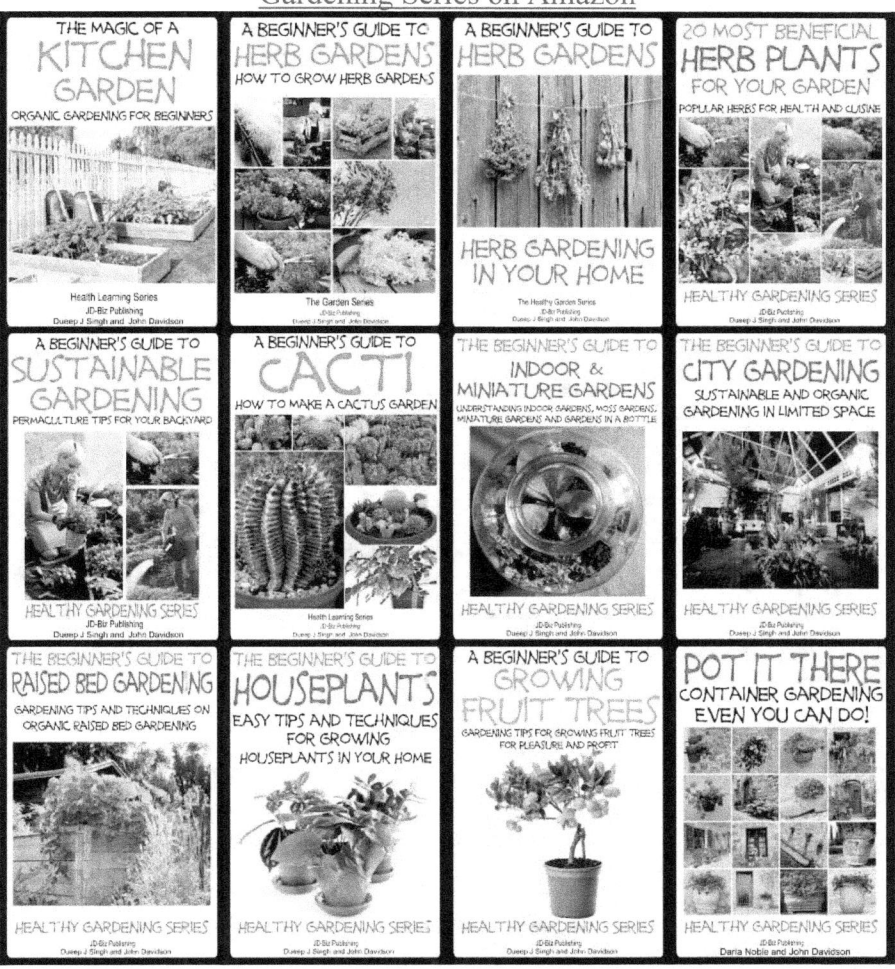

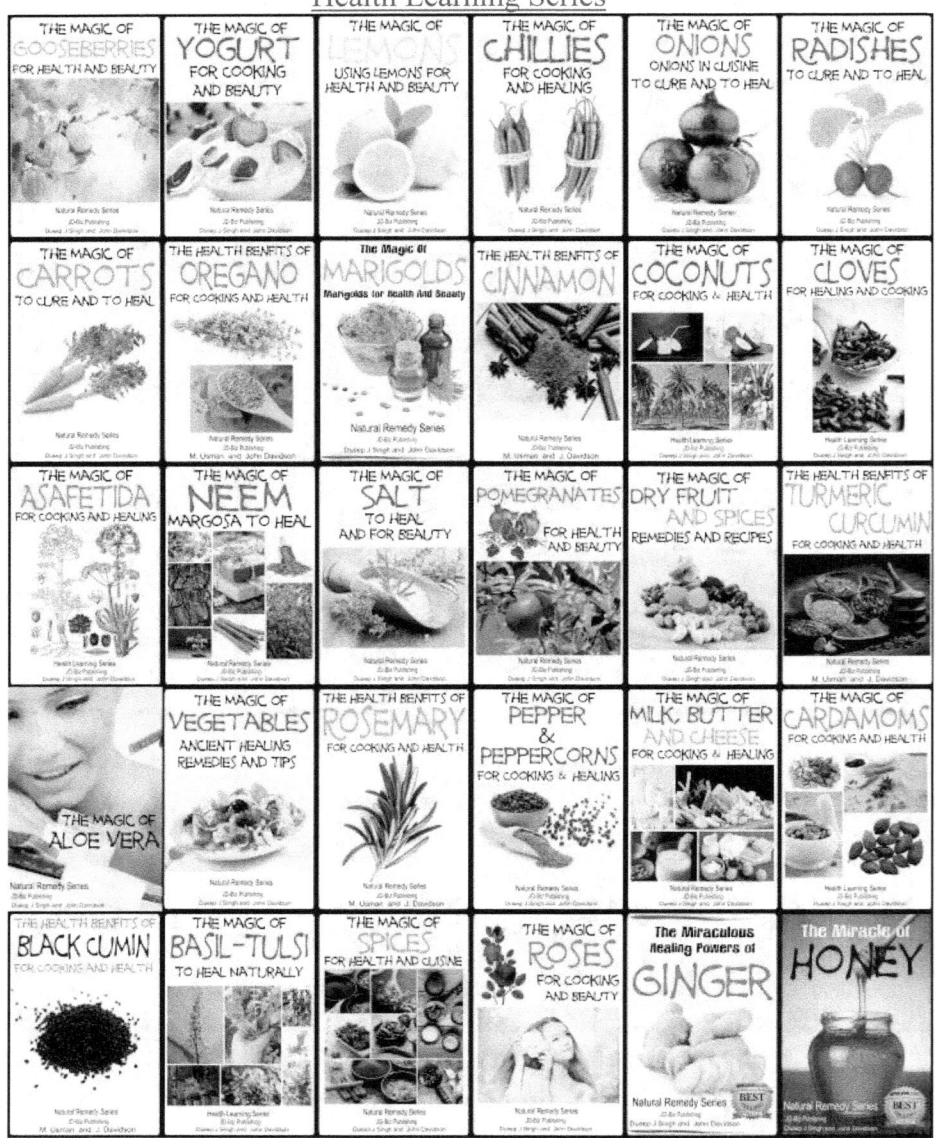

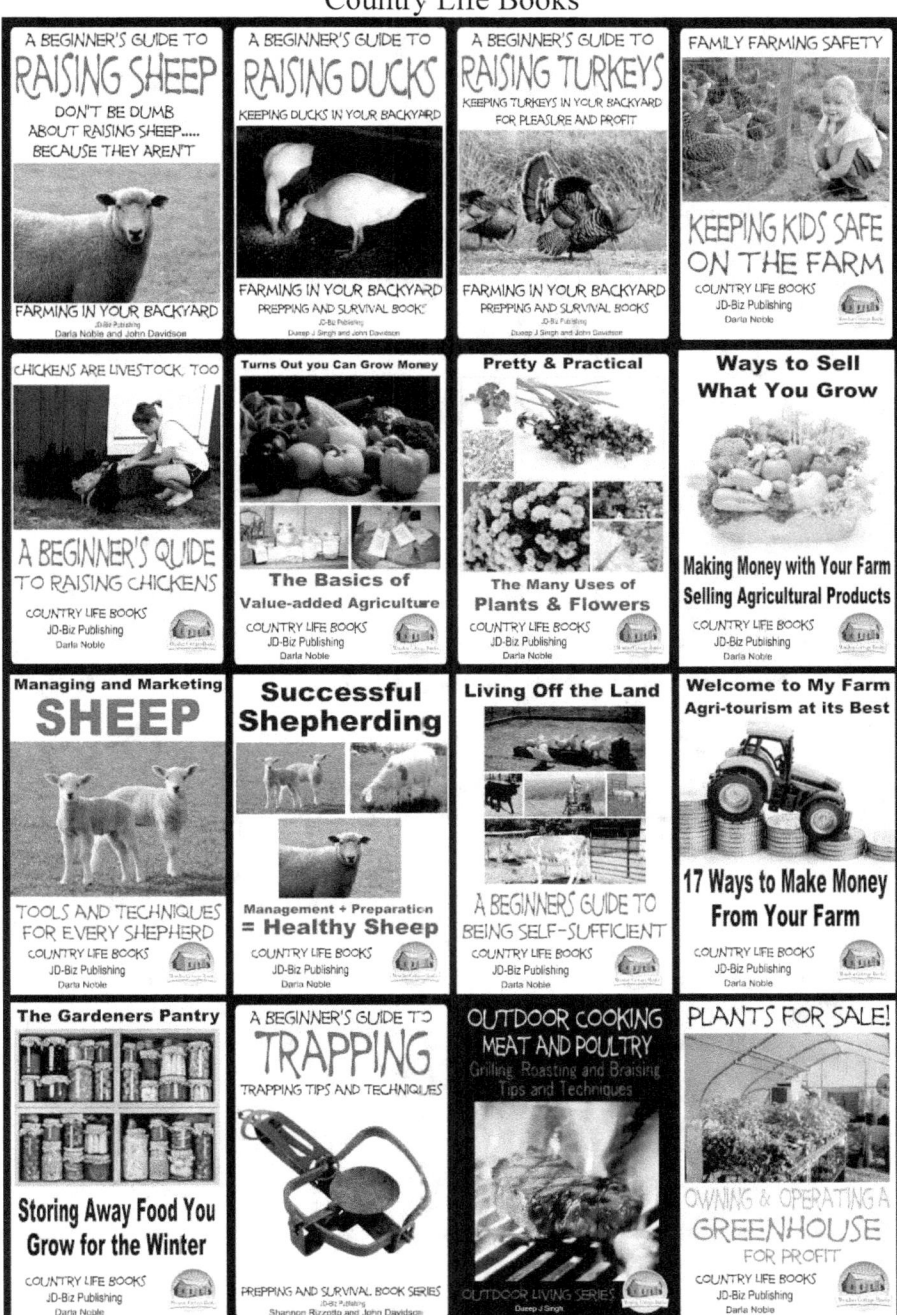

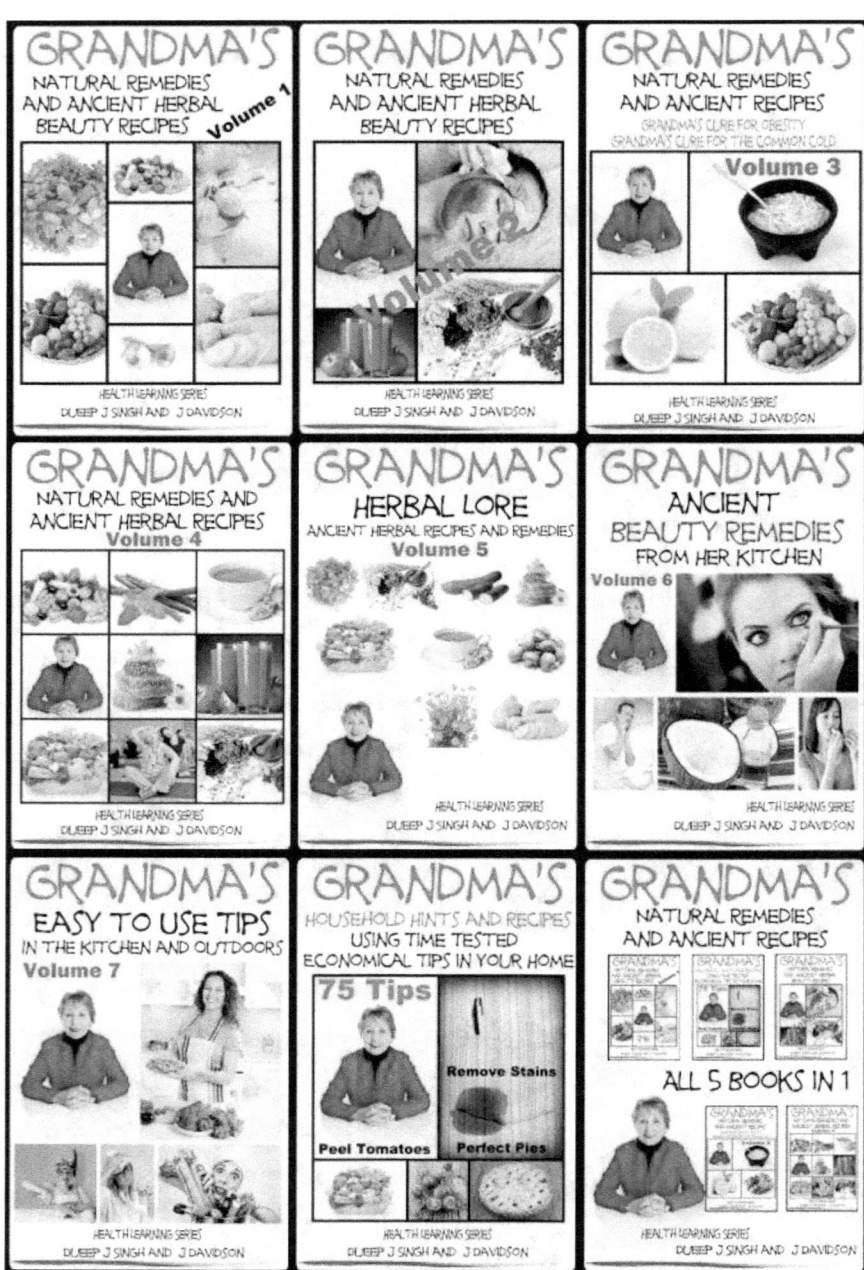

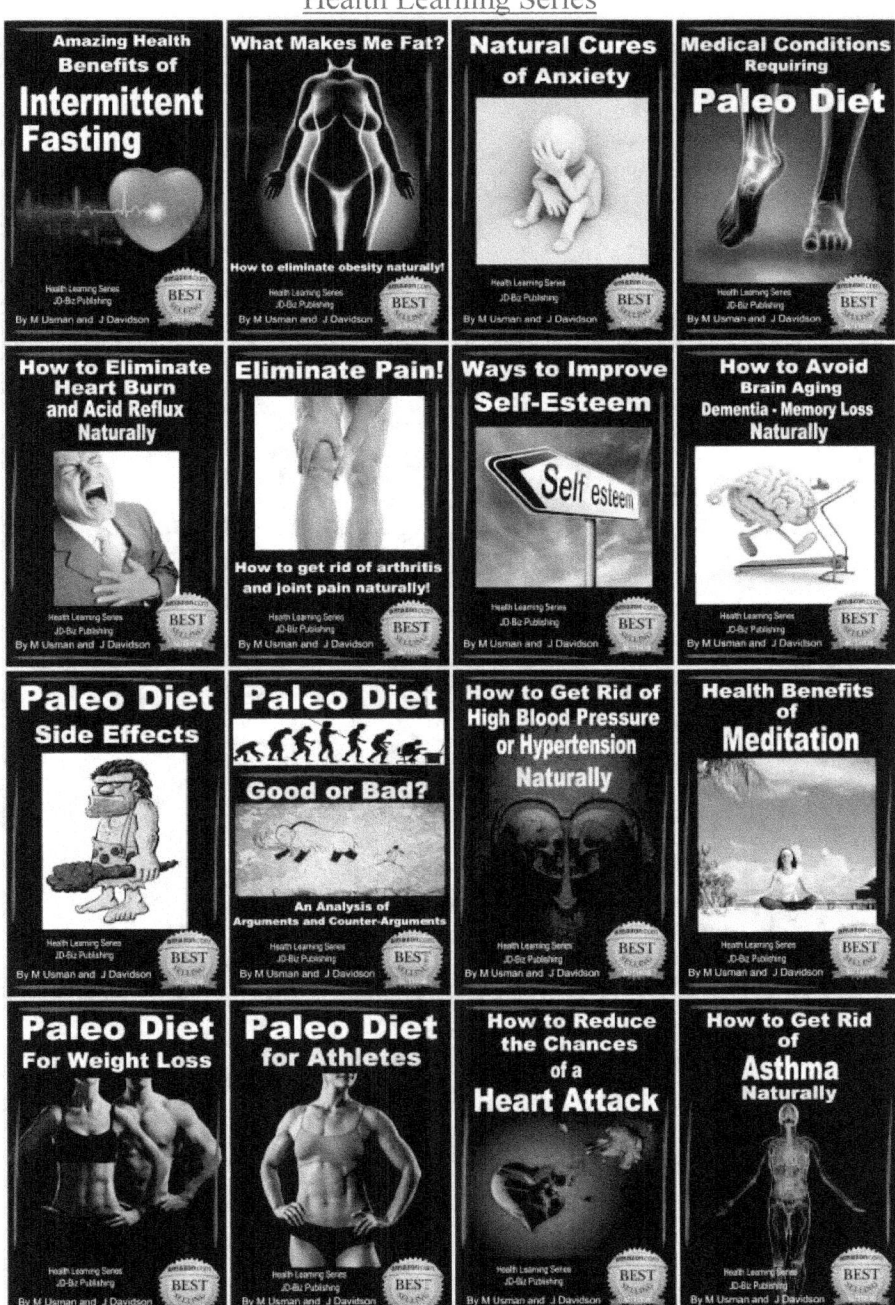

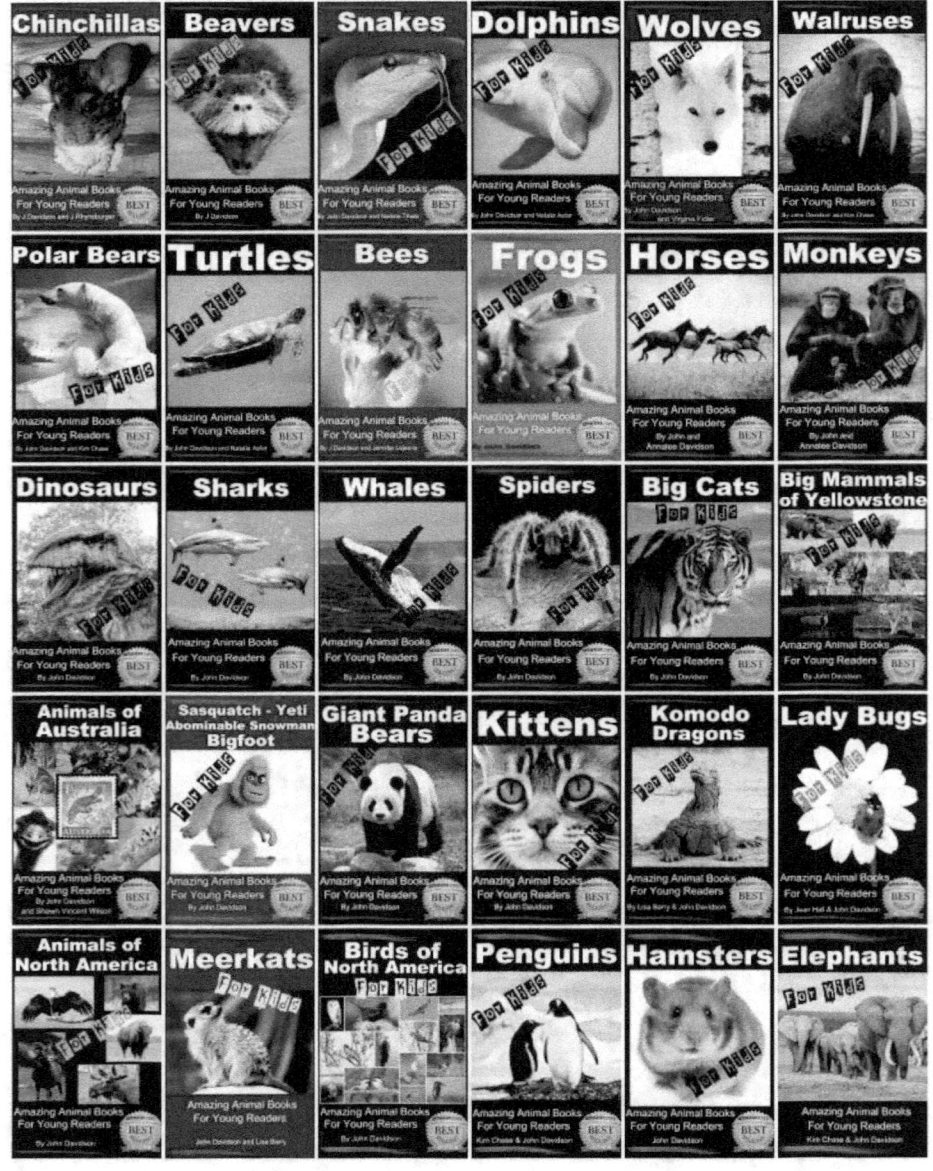

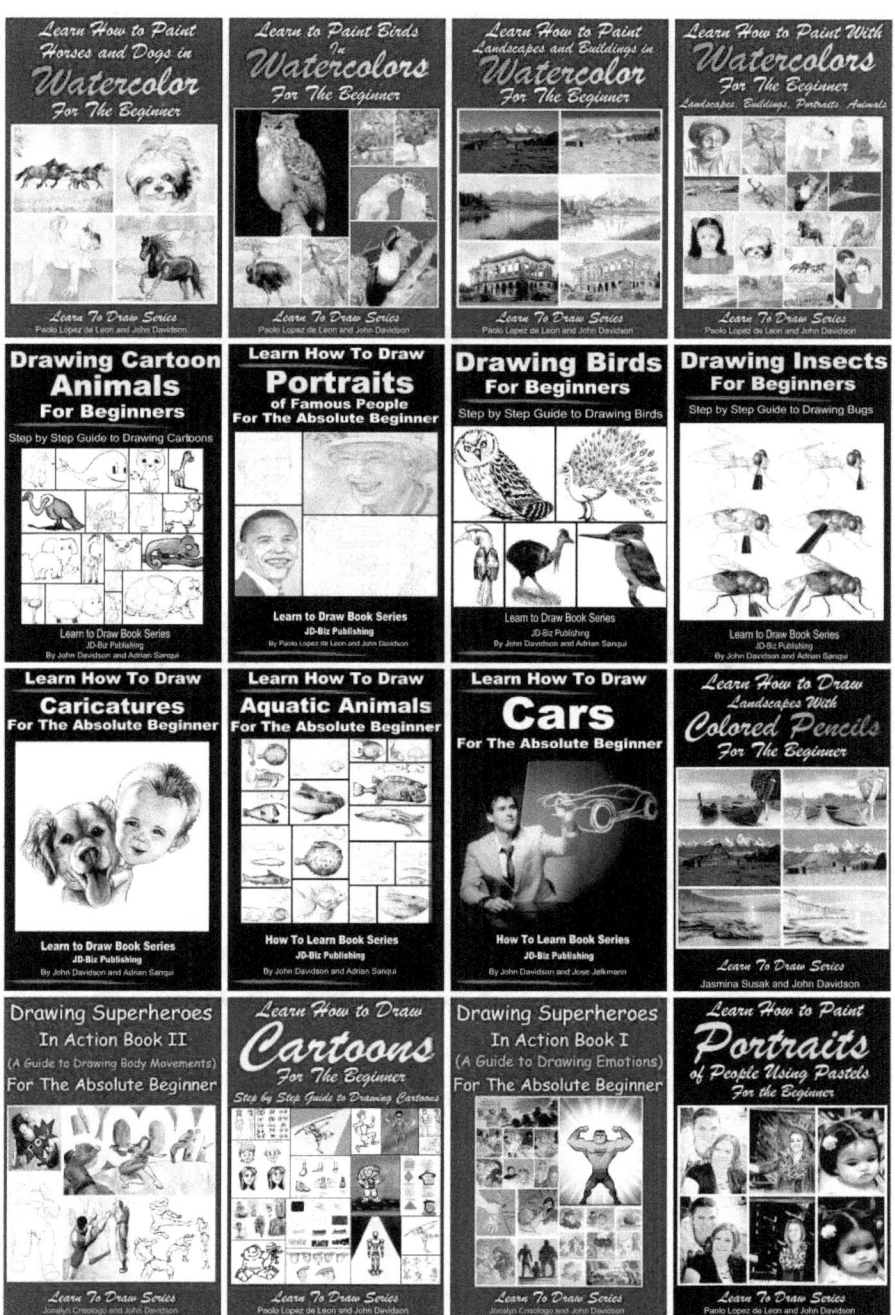

How to Build and Plan Books

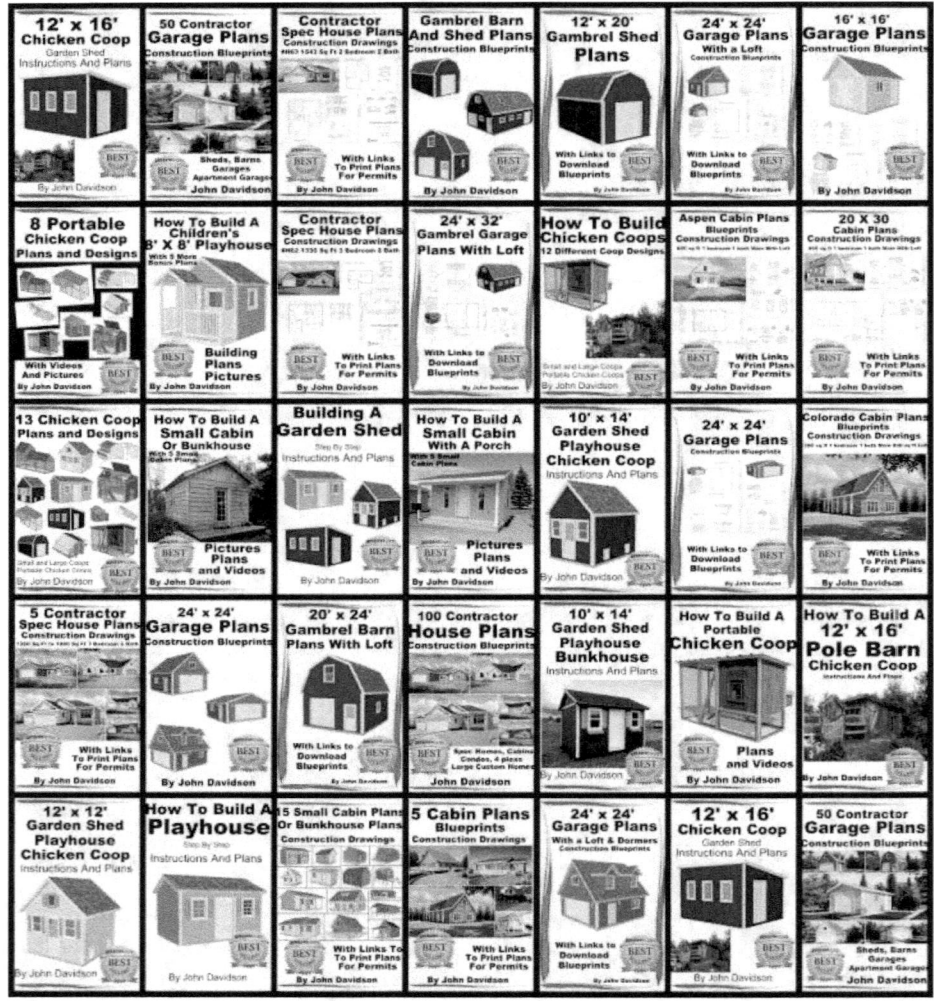

Entrepreneur Book Series

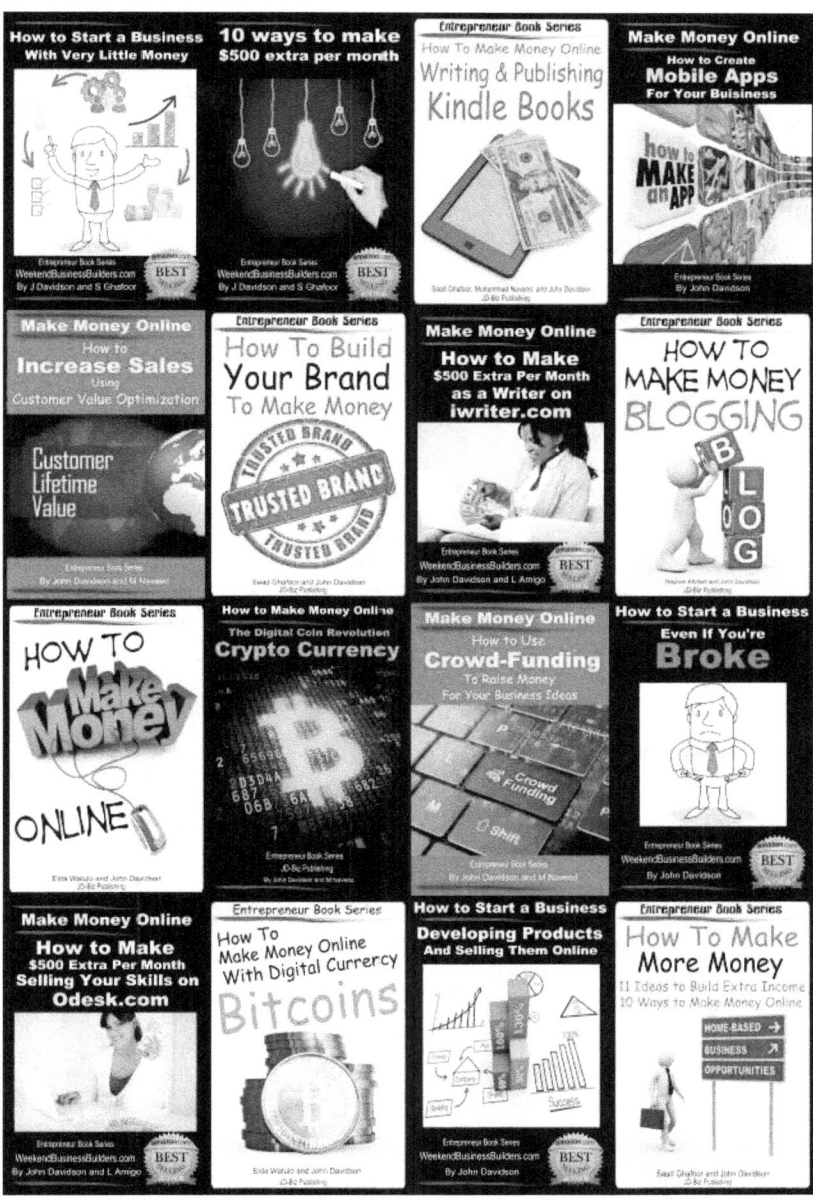

Our books are available at

1. Amazon.com
2. Barnes and Noble
3. Itunes
4. Kobo
5. Smashwords
6. Google Play Books

Download Free Books!

http://MendonCottageBooks.com

Publisher

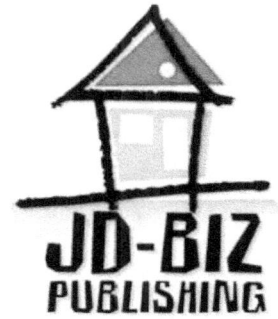

JD-Biz Corp

P O Box 374

Mendon, Utah 84325

http://www.jd-biz.com/

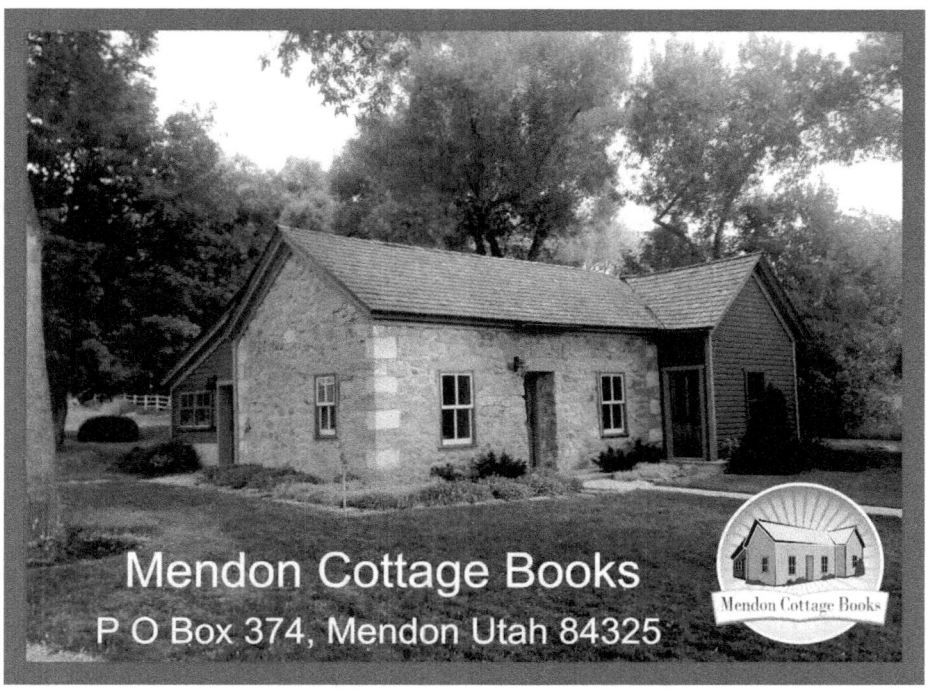

www.ingramcontent.com/pod-product-compliance
Lightning Source LLC
Chambersburg PA
CBHW061929280526
45787CB00004B/1536